BRANDY AND SALT - THE ULTIMATE MEDICINE?

OLD THERAPY OF WILLIAM LEE FROM 1850 REDISCOVERED

JAMIE WILD

ISBN 978-1-63920-215-7

Contents

Preface   *v*

  1. What Is Brandy   1

  2. Health Benefits Of Brandy   4

  3. French Brandy   7

  4. About Salt   12

  5. Health Benefits Of Salt   16

  6. Brandy And Salt (the Perfect Remedy)   19

  7. Diseases And Mode Of Treatment.   22

  8. Conclusion   38

Preface

The in?uiry has often been made of me whether gin, rum, or spirits of wine, will not do as well as brandy, or if British brandy is not as good as French brandy. With regard to the first three, gin, rum, or spirits of wine, I should recommend all such to make the experiment for themselves ; for myself, I have always been content with French brandy. But with regard to whether British brandy is as good as French brandy.

There was an occurrence which took place in a neighboring town in this county: Two gentlemen, from the perusal of one of my letters in the Intelligencer, agreed to make use of the remedy, for the same complaint; I believe, the rheumatism.

They mixed and used it according to the prescription. After a few days they compared notes, when it was found that one of them was almost cured, whilst the other was not at all better.

They then spoke of the manner they had mixed and used it, of the kind of brandy, when it came out that the one cured used French brandy, and the other British brandy.

CHAPTER ONE

WHAT IS BRANDY

Brandy is an alcoholic beverage that has been around in some form or another for centuries. The name brandy actually comes from a Dutch word "brandewijn" and is made by further distilling wine to increase the alcoholic content.The distillation of wine has been occurring since Classic times, but it was not widely understood or propagated until the 15th century. This form of li?uor is typically between 30-60% alcohol by volume, which can pack ?uite a punch when drunk in excess. However, brandy is usually enjoyed as an after-dinner drink, not as something that one drinks all evening, as you may do with wine or beer at a party.

Brandy is derived from wine, yet it is aged in oak barrels, which increases the alcohol content and also gives it the uni?ue color.Brandy enjoys some of the same health benefits as wine, although most people are unaware of them. Many people think of alcoholic beverages as inherent vices, something that is very enjoyable, but can also punish you with hangovers, empty wallets, diseased livers, and addiction. As can be said of anything from sugar to red wine – everything in moderation!brandy

Grapes are the defacto standard fruit for brandy but many types of fruits including apples, peaches, plums, pears, or cherries can be used. If the fruit is anything other than grape, it must be marked on the label.

Brandy is fre?uently aged in oak casks that help mellow the flavor and adds additional aromas and flavor from the wood itself. Brandy that is aged less than two years is called 'immature' or unaged brandy and an age statement is required on the label. Brandy that is aged over two years is considered 'mature' and may or may not contain an age statement on the label.

Some brandies, are aged using the solera system, where the producer changes the barrel each year. After a period of aging, which depends on the style, class and legal requirements, the mature brandy is mixed with distilled water to reduce alcohol concentration and bottled. The final brandy is generally reduced to 70 – 120 proof.

Many countries have their own version of brandy that come from a specific geographic location like Cognac that comes from the Cognac region of France or Armagnac that comes from the Armagnac region in Gascony, southwest France.

Brandy is much the same, and while it does fall into the category of "hard alcohol", it is produced in a uni?ue way, is composed of interesting substances, and therefore offers different benefits and effects, as compared to other types of alcohol. As many people assume that alcohol only harms health, it is important to do your due diligence and see how there's nothing wrong with enjoying a drink or two from time to time, particularly if its as beneficial as brandy! Let's take a closer look at some of the important health benefits of brandy.

How to take brandy?

Brandy is a strong alcohol spirit that is made from fermented fruit juice or wine. Although it is not as popular as it once was, brandy remains a popular choice for those looking for high-?uality alcohol. Some other common names for brandy are applejack and cognac. Brandy comes in many different varieties, based on different fruits, and can be purchased in many different price ranges. Typically, it is considered an after-dinner drink.

Brandy can be drunk in any manner you see fit, but the popular ways are to pour it neat (without ice) into a snifter, which is held in the hand, so the glass can be warmed. This will release more of the aroma of the brandy, and makes for a more enjoyable drink. Brandy is something that should be sipped, starting with small sips and gradually growing larger. You should also try to inhale the aroma of the brandy as you drink it. Cocktails are also an option, but only with less expensive brandy.

Is brandy whiskey?

Brandy is not a type of whiskey but many people may mistake brandy for whiskey, due to the similar burning sensation of drinking it. Brandy is primarily made from wine and fermented fruit juices, whereas to classify as whiskey, the spirit must be made from a type of grain, such as wheat, corn or malted barley. They both may sting your chest on the way down, but they are two very different types of alcohol.

CHAPTER TWO

HEALTH BENEFITS OF BRANDY

Heart Health: As with many different types of alcohol, brandy can have an effect on the heart. When drunk in moderation, research has shown that brandy contains a wide range of beneficial antioxidants, much like the wine from which it is derived. This antioxidant potential can actually reduce the amount of negative cholesterol in the heart, helping to balance out cholesterol levels and reducing pla?ue build-up.

Preventing atherosclerosis is one of the best ways to avoid the potentially disastrous effects of heart attacks and strokes. Furthermore, the polyphenolic compounds in brandy significantly reduce inflammation in the cardiovascular system, which eases tension in the blood vessels and lowers blood pressure.

However, as with any type of alcohol, drinking excessive amounts can also be bad for the heart, so caution should always be taken when monitoring consumption. A single glass after dinner is recommended as a safe and beneficial amount.

Anti-Aging Capacity: The antioxidant compounds found in brandy, some of which are attributed to the presence of copper in some of the aging barrels, can have a strong effect on the body. Antioxidants are organic compounds and substances that eliminate free radicals in our body or neutralize their effects.

Free radicals are the dangerous byproducts of cellular metabolism that can cause our body's healthy cells to mutate or undergo apoptosis (cell death). Antioxidants can help prevent this type of cellular death in the skin, hair, internal organs, and brain, among many others. Therefore, brandy has been shown to effectively prevent certain types of aging symptoms, including wrinkles on the skin, cognitive issues, poor vision, and other chronic conditions that occur as we age.

Cancer Treatment: Although there are certain cancers that are exacerbated by excessive li?uor consumption, brandy has been connected to the treatment or prevention of certain cancers. One of the essential components of brandy is ellagic acid, which is a powerful organic compound that can prevent the development and spread of cancerous cells. This is most obviously seen with bladder and ovarian cancer, but this area of research is an exciting new area that may increase brandy's importance as a healthy li?uor choice for people. This is accomplished by the activation of a certain gene (by ellagic acid) that inhibits growth and metastasis of cancerous cells!

Sleep Issues: When it comes to alcohol helping you sleep, most people think of drinking too much alcohol and dozing off; however, brandy also has certain soothing, warming, and relaxing qualities that can help to induce healthy, restful sleep. Granted, the high alcohol content will also help the system due to its natural depressant ?ualities, which is one of the reasons that brandy is often suggested as an after-dinner drink, in preparation for sleep.

Weight Issues: Unlike carbohydrate-heavy alcoholic drinks, like beer, brandy contains no carbs and doesn't fill you up. Brandy can also be enjoyed as an aperitif, without ruining your appetite, nor does it contribute to the simple sugar breakdown of carbs that can easily be stored as fat, such as those found in beer.

Respiratory Conditions: Traditionally, brandy has been used as an effective means to relieve respiratory issues, such as coughs or sore throats. The strong alcoholic content can help eliminate bacteria and loosens up phlegm and mucus, thereby acting as a type of expectorant. The anti-inflammatory properties in brandy can also help soothe the irritation that causes coughing and sore throats.

Immune System: For hundreds of years, brandy has been relied on as a traditional solution for the common cold or flu. The natural warming properties of brandy, mixed with its relaxing quality that induces healthy sleep and the antibacterial nature of alcohol, all make this popular and delicious li?uor a popular boost for the immune system. It can eliminate pathogens that may be in your system and can boost your immune system with the help of its antioxidants.

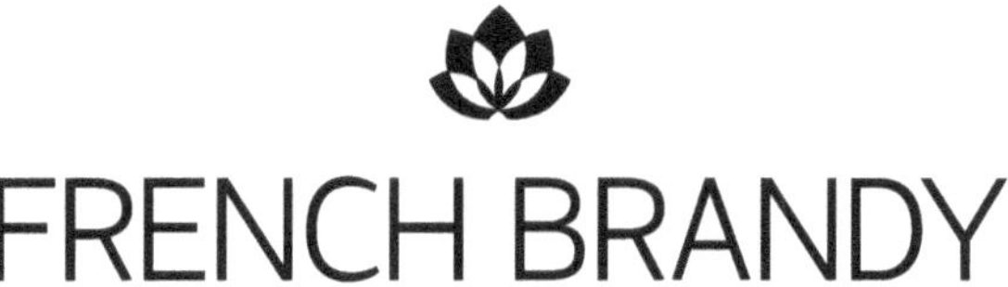

CHAPTER THREE

FRENCH BRANDY

French brandies are made from the wine of the St. Émillion, Colombard (or Folle Blanche) grapes. However, anything that will ferment can be distilled and turned into a brandy. Grapes, apples, blackberries, sugar cane, honey, milk, rice, wheat, corn, potatoes, and rye are all commonly fermented and distilled. In a time of shortage, desperate people will substitute anything to have access to alcohol.

The first step in making fine brandies is to allow the fruit juice (typically grape) to ferment. This usually means placing the juice, or must as it is known in the distilling trade, in a large vat at 68-77°F (20-25°C) and leaving it for five days. During this period, natural yeast present in the distillery environment will ferment the sugar present in the must into alcohol and carbon dioxide. The white wine grapes used for most fine brandy usually ferment to an alcohol content of around 10%.

Fine brandies are always made in small batches using pot stills. A pot still is simply a large pot, usually made out of copper, with a bulbous top. The pot still is heated to the point where the fermented li?uid reaches the boiling point of alcohol. The alcohol vapors, which contain a large amount of water vapor, rise in the still into the bulbous top.

The vapors are funneled from the pot still through a bent pipe to a condenser where the vapors are chilled, condensing the vapors back to a liquid with a much higher alcohol content. The purpose of the bulbous top and bent pipe is to allow undesirable compounds to condense and fall back into the still. Thus, these elements do not end up in the final product.

Most fine brandy makers double distill their brandy, meaning they concentrate the alcohol twice. It takes about 9 gal (34 1) of wine to make I gal (3.8 1) of brandy. After the first distillation, which takes about eight hours, 3,500 gal (13,249 1) of wine have been converted to about 1,200 gal (4,542 1) of concentrated li?uid (not yet brandy) with an alcohol content of 26-32%. The French limit the second distillation (la bonne chauffe) to batches of 660 gal (2,498 1). The product of the second distillation has an alcohol content of around 72%. The higher the alcohol content the more neutral (tasteless) the brandy will be. The lower the alcohol content, the more of the underlying flavors will remain in the brandy, but there is a much greater chance that off flavors will also make their way into the final product.

The brandy is not yet ready to drink after the second distillation. It must first be placed in oak casks and allowed to age, an important step in the production process. Most brandy consumed today, even fine brandy, is less than six years old. However, some fine brandies are more than 50 years old. As the brandy ages, it absorbs flavors from the oak while its own structure softens, becoming less astringent. Through evaporation, brandy will lose about 1% of its alcohol per year for the first 50 years or so it is "on oak."

Fine brandy can be ready for bottling after two years, some after six years, and some not for decades. Some French cognacs are alleged to be from the time of Napoleon. However, these claims are unlikely to be true. A ploy used by the cognac makers is to continually remove 90% of the cognac from an old barrel and then refill it with younger brandy. It does not take many repetitions of this tactic to dilute any trace of the Napoleonic-age brandy.

Fine brandies are usually blended from many different barrels over a number of vintages. Some cognacs can contain brandy from up to a 100 different barrels. Because most brandies have not spent 50 years in the barrel, which would naturally reduce their alcohol contents to the traditional 40%, the blends are diluted with distilled water until they reach the proper alcohol content. Sugar, to simulate age in young brandies, is added along with a little caramel to obtain a uniform color consistency across the entire production run. The resulting product can cost anywhere from $25 to $500 or even more for very rare brandy.

Mass-produced brandy

Mass-produced brandy, other than having the same alcohol content, has very little in common with fine brandy. Both start with wine, though the mass-produced brandies are likely to be made from table grape varieties like the Thompson Seedless rather than from fine wine grapes. Instead of the painstaking double distillation in small batches, mass-produced brandies are made via fractional distillation in column stills. Column stills are sometimes called continuous stills as raw material is continuously poured into the top while the final product and wastes continuously come out of the side and bottom.

A column still is about 30-ft (9-m) high and contains a series of horizontal, hollow baffles that are interconnected. Hot wine is poured into the top of the column while steam is run through the hollow baffles; the steam and wine do not mix directly. The alcohol and other low boiling point liquids in the wine evaporate. The vapors rise while the non-alcoholic liquids fall. As the still is cooler at the top, the rising vapors eventually get to a part of the still where they will condense, each type of vapor at a temperature just above its own boiling point.

The distillation of brandy.

Once they have recondensed, the liquids begin to move downward in the still. As they fall, they boil again. This process of boiling and condensing, rising and falling, happens over and over again in the column. The various components of the wine fraction and collect in the column where the temperature is just below the boiling point of that component.

This allows the ethyl alcohol condensate to be bled out of the column at the height where it collects. The resulting product is a pure spirit, colorless, odorless, and tasteless, with an alcohol content of about 96.5%. At 96.5% alcohol, it can be used to fuel automobiles. It can be diluted and called vodka or diluted and flavored with juniper berries and called gin.

Mass-produced brandies are also aged in oak casks and pick up some flavors from them. Like its fine counterpart, the brandies are blended, diluted to around 40% alcohol, and bottled.

• 11 •

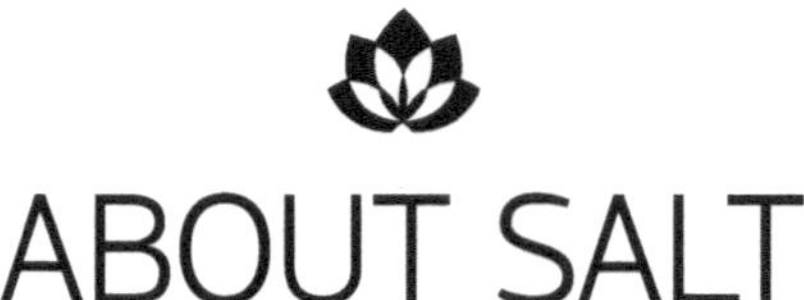

ABOUT SALT

We all need salt, and we get it from many sources; our food, sea food, and "table salt". We are told that sea salt and table salt have the same nutritional value. So what is the difference, and does it matter?

The real differences between sea salt and table salt are in their taste and texture.Sea salt is harvested from seawater through evaporation. Table salt is harvested from mineral deposits. Unfortunately, both types of salt can be refined, resulting in pure sodium chloride.

Table salt is a fine-grained salt that can contain added iodine which is necessary for normal thyroid function, and can also contain anti-caking ingredients. It may have been harvested mechanically from with bulldozers and bagged or piped into transport containers, and they processed to remove contaminates. Unfortunately this process may also remove nutrients beneficial to us.

Sea salt is available in packets, or grinders, coarse or fine ground, bleached, or unprocessed. Some people prefer sea salt to table salt because they claim it has a more subtle flavor, and some people use sea salt because they believe it has more minerals....and it may do, if it hasn't been bleached, or had minerals removed to make more profit in other areas.

Natural Salt is an essential element in the diet of not only humans but of animals, and animals will travel to use their "salt lick». The use of natural salt is as old as human history. Natural Salt is one of the most effective and most widely used of all food seasonings and natural preservatives. Natural salt is a source of 21 essential and 30 accessory minerals that are essential to our health.

Natural gray sea salts of which Celtic Sea Salts are one, have been harvested by natural means, and claims to be unprocessed. This soft grey salt contributes both flavor and nutrients to the food we use, replenishing and helping to balance our electrolyte system. The 82 vital trace minerals give all our systems the minerals they need for optimal function.

Our journey through history has revealed that the antiseptic action of salt on the skin and mucous membranes has been known for a very long time. Scientific studies have now confirmed the effectiveness of salt therapy in several indications. The antiseptic and bactericidal ?ualities of dental salt (sea salt) help remove pla?ue which is a cause of gingivitis and caries. Salt is being increasingly used as support treatment for skin diseases.

Chronically inflamed skin is treated with medical bath salt from the Dead Sea (d) or table salt. The salt peels off dandruff, reduces inflammation, itching and pain, and helps regenerate the skin. Salt-baths are fre?uently used to treat psoriasis, atopic dermatitis, chronic eczema as well as arthritis. Sometimes (as in psoriasis), this therapy is followed by ultraviolet light radiotherapy under strict medical control so that the combination of salt water and UV light does not expose patients to an increased risk of skin cancer.

The ancient Greeks had already recommended seaside health resorts to cure skin diseases and Paracelsus mentioned the effectiveness of "salt brine". Sea-water baths later led to salt-water baths in regions closely linked with the extraction of salt (salt mines, springs and works) but it was not until 1800 that doctors from the German town of Bad Nauheim introduced a methodical salt-bath therapy (6). They tried to obtain scientific evidence for claims regarding the healing effects of the waters.

Current medical indications for salt-bath therapy rest, as a matter of principle, on the empirical traditions of centuries. They include support treatment for skin diseases due to the anti-inflammatory action of salt. Patients suffering from rheumatic conditions often experience relief from joint pain when moving about in a salt bath.

Finally, common or Dead Sea salt can be used as an additive especially in body care products (ointments, shampoos, gels, washes and body lotions).

Inhaling salt

Steam from salt water is inhaled in chronic diseases of the upper and lower respiratory track (pharynx, paranasal sinuses, and bronchial tree) or to ease the discomfort of a common cold. Let's not forget that Hippocrates had already recommended this treatment! The age-old method is to heat a salt solution to obtain steam but modern ultrasound atomising can now transport minute salt particles directly to tiny bronchia. The main effects of salt on the bronchial system are to stimulate secretion, loosen and help eliminate viscous secretions, inhibit inflammation, reduce irritation causing cough, clean the mucous membrane of the kinocilium, and contract (bronchoconstriction) or extend (dilatation) the respiratory ducts.

Drinking salt water

Salt water when drunk has an expectorant effect in the stomach and increases gastric juice secretion. It raises the level of stomach acid, hastens its production, impedes or stimulates stomach motricity and emptying-rate (depending upon the salt concentration), increases the secretion of the pancreas, and at higher salt concentrations stimulates the formation of bile acids.

CHAPTER FIVE

HEALTH BENEFITS OF SALT

Sore throats, toothaches, postnasal drip, bee stings, mosquito bites, painful gums, poison ivy, and poison oak are some of the ailments for which salt has been prescribed. Modern science doesn't endorse all of the traditional uses of salt, but this article offers a picture of the seemingly endless healing ?ualities salt may have.

Sore Throat: The simplest remedy for minor sore throat pain is a warm saltwater gargle (no matter how much you dislike the taste!). Just add 1 teaspoon salt to 8 ounces warm water, and gargle several times a day. See a physician if the sore throat persists longer than 3 days or is accompanied by a high fever.

Burns or Injuries: A severe burn in your mouth from eating something very hot can be relieved by rinsing with saltwater every hour or so. Use 1/2 teaspoon salt in 8 ounces warm water.

Biting the tongue or cheek can result in a large amount of blood but is rarely serious. To help ease the pain, rinse mouth with 1 teaspoon salt in 1 cup warm water.

Gums: Swish with 1 teaspoon salt in 4 ounces warm water when gums are painful. If you have an abscess, the salt will draw out some of the infection. Any gum pain should be treated by a dentist as soon as possible.

Toothaches: As a temporary remedy for a toothache before going to the dentist, rinse your mouth with a mixture of 4 ounces warm water, 2 tablespoons vinegar, and 1 tablespoon salt.

Add 1/4 teaspoon salt and 1/4 teaspoon baking soda to 8 ounces warm (not hot) water. Gargle with the mixture 3 times a day to ease your sore throat. If pain persists longer than 3 days, contact a physician.

Nose: Make your own saline nose drops to use for controlling annoying postnasal drip. People with sleep apnea, a condition that involves a dangerous interruption of breathing while asleep, may also want to try these drops to help keep nasal passages open.

Bee stings and bug bites: Work a mixture of salt and water into a paste that will stick to a bee sting or bug bite. Apply the paste, and let sit until dry. This should relieve any itch or pain.Combine equal parts baking soda and salt, then brush onto a sting or bite area to help relieve itch.

Treat a mosquito bite by soaking it for a few minutes in saltwater, then applying an ointment made of salt and lard.

Poison ivy and poison oak: Help poison ivy clear up more ?uickly by soaking irritated skin in hot saltwater.

Allergies: Irrigating the nostrils and sinuses with saltwater is an excellent way to control persistent, annoying allergy symptoms. Dissolve 1/2 teaspoon salt in 8 ounces room temperature water. Draw mixture into a nose dropper, and inhale li?uid through your nostrils. Repeat several times for each nostril, using 2 or 3 drops of the solution each time. When you are through, blow your nose until no discharge remains.

CHAPTER SIX

BRANDY AND SALT (THE PERFECT REMEDY)

Half fill a bottle with brandy, and add to it one third the ?uantity of salt; cork and shake well together. When mixed, let the salt settle to the bottom, and be particularly careful to use it when clear, the clearer the better. Many persons have made a great mistake in shaking it up just before it is used.

The efficacy is not near so great, and to open sores the application is much more painful, from the particles of salt which are not dissolved in the brandy ; but the salt and brandy should remain together, and when all the brandy is used oil' more may be added to the salt. Though it is ready for use in twenty minutes after it is put together, it is good at any time after; and nit is a perfect medicine, as it has the rare ?uality of being greatly nefficacious in either internal or external application.

GENERAL RULES TO BE OBSERVED IN USING THE REMEDY.

Begin with taking one table-spoonful, mixed in a little hot water or tea, an hour before breakfast, and gradually increase, if the stomach will bear it, to two. The remedy must always betaken in water as hot as the patient can drink it, except in cases of worms and paralytic attacks, and in those two cases to be taken pure.

For children from two to ten years of age, one half of the ?uantity here prescribed will be sufficient, and increase it according to the age above those years. In all cases where the head'is directed to be rubbed, it should be done so all over, from the back to the front, and the hair made very wet, with the remedy pure ; the more hair the better. The operation should be continued for ten minutes or a ?uarter of an hour before going to bed, and the head should then be covered with the cap only.

For pain in any part of the body except the head, bind the parts affected with linen saturated with the remedy. Abstinence from Intoxicating Drinks. To insure success it is absolutely necessary that, during its application, whether internally or externally, the patient should strictly abstain from all stimulating and exciting drinks, except the Brandy and Salt. This is a rule which can never be departed from with safety.

Opening Medicine. — The bowels must, be kept open at all times, but especially when the patient is using the remedy. The kind of opening medicine which I recommend and use myself, as I find it answers best, is the following: — Four ounces of Epsom salts, dissolved in half a pint of hot water; then add half a pint of cold water and one tea-spoonful of the essence of peppermint. A wine-glassful to be taken when re?uired, on going to bed. It is better to add half a table-spoonful of brandy to each dose.

I found it very efficacious to wet a piece of fine linen with the remedy, and bind it on my leg, which I kept moist by pouring a few drops on the linen ; the more frequently I did so the better. This I strictly attended to for about three weeks, and though my leg had been very bad for many months, and bid defiance to the best medical aid I could procure, which caused me to give up all hopes of recovery, to my great surprise the inflammation was entirely gone, the wounds healed, and the leg well in a month.

CHAPTER SEVEN

DISEASES AND MODE OF TREATMENT.

Dizziness in the Head is cured by washing the crown of the head with the remedy pure. It ought to be rubbed for half an hour, even when the dizzinc; is removed. Sometimes it feels cured during the operation; sometimes in an hour after; and even it has not been removed until after retiring to "bed.

There are instances of this complaint returning several times, but it is easily subdued by the manner of appbying this remedy. Determination of Blood to the Head, which, by the regular mode of practice is sought to be cured by bleeding with leeches about the temples, though it does not always cure, generally, brings the patient to the borders of the grave.

This complaint is greatly abated, and very often cured, by rubbing the crown of the head with the remedy. Sometimes it is removed very soon, and generally by one operation; if not, it may be repeated once, in which case it is necessary that the afflicted should take two table-spoonsful of the remedy, diluted with six or eight table-spoonsful of hot water. The rubbing of the head is always the best on retiring to bed, and the dose, should be taken in the morning, about an hour before breakfast, and repeated several times.

Headaches are removed by rubbing the head with the remedy, in the same manner as for Determination of Blood to the Head. I have applied it in hundreds of instances, and always with success; but in case the Headache proves obstinate, it should be repealed, and two table-spoonsful, with six or eight table-spoonsful of hot water, should be taken ; but it is generally cured by rubbing once.

Inflammation in the Eyes. —this remedy, if it only cured this complaint in the manner it does, is beyond all price. There is no occa-sion for dark rooms ; no occasion to desist from the ordinary occupations of the afflicted ; no cauterizing of the eye, which very often causes the afflicted to lose their sight ; no distress in families. It is cured by the patient wetting the corner of his handkerchief five or six times each clay, with the remedy, pure, when be is at his work, when he is walking, when he is riding, when he is buying or selling his merchandize; and rubbing it each time well into his eve.

The pain is very trifling, and the cure certain. How different this is from the usual treatment. A friend of mine, was shut up in a dark room for ten weeks. He had his eye cauterized several times, besides having several operations performed upon him, and after all his eye is not so well cured as it would have been by this remedy in a fortnight, if it had been taken in time; but in that case he perhaps would have said the inflammation was not severe.

Inflammation of the Eyes. — The eye to be bathed two or three times a day with a portion of the remedy diluted in an equal quantity of water. If the eye be much inflamed, add a white bread poultice on going to bed, placed between two cloths.

Inflammation in the Brain is cured by rubbing the crown of the head with the remedy until the pain is removed. There are several instances in which very valuable lives might have been prolonged by the use of this remedy. Malibran, whilst at Manchester, fell a sacrifice to it ; and I am confident that if it had been applied as above, her life would have been spared.

Toothache is cured in a manner which I discovered myself. It is simply by filling the ear on that side of the head where the pain is with the remedy pure, and letting it remain in the ear for ten minutes, in most cases sufficient to remove the pain. I have seldom known it fail. For any other than decayed teeth the cure is generally permanent. For decayed teeth it may return again upon taking cold; it should remain in the ear from five to ten minutes.

Earache is cured the same as the Toothache, by filling the ear with the remedy. This is rather a pleasant operation, and calculated to do great good in other respects.

Deafness is greatly relieved, and very often cured, by the same method, filling the ear with the remedy. I have known it to be of great use in several instances; and since I have filled my ears with it I can hear with greater clearness. The best time is upon retiring to rest. Fill first the ear which is the least affected with deafness, and let it remain in for ten minutes; after which fill the other ear, and let it remain in the ear all night. It conduces very much to sound sleeping.

Teeth are preserved by putting a little of the remedy, once each week or fortnight, upon the tooth brush when it is used. This will also remove any soreness which may be in the teeth from eating sour fruit, or any other cause.

Gum BotLS are cured by saturating a piece of fine linen with the remedy, and applying it to the part, betwixt the gums and the cheek. The best time is upon retiring to rest, and letting it remain the whole, of the night; this will remove the most violent pain. But the same operation re?uires to be repeated several nights to remove the boil and prevent the teeth from becoming loose.

Eruptions upon the Face and Head are generally removed by rubbing the part with the remedy. If they are of a cancerous nature, and of a few weeks' standing, the remedy gives no pain, and the cure is effected with surprising facility; but to all other descriptions of eruptions it gives pain.

Ague, or Intermitting Fevers, are cured by rubbing the head once, on retiring to rest, and next morning taking two tablespoonsful, diluted with six table-spoonsful of hot water for a man, and half the quantity for a female, an hour before breakfast. It should be repeated for twelve mornings, or until the disorder is subdued.

Cholic is generally cured in four or five minutes, by taking two table-spoonsful of the remedy, diluted with hot water. If it is not cured by the first operation, it ought to be repeated, and the dose made stronger. It seldom re?uires repeating more than twice, though I have known it repeated three times.

Cholera is cured by rubbing the head once or twice, or as often as the pains in the head return, and by taking two or three table-spoonsful, diluted with hot water. This should be repeated several times each day, if the attack is very strong, at short intervals; and if the skin is discolored, the part ought to be rubbed with it until the complaint is subdued, which will be known by the removal of the pain.

Quinsey, or Sore Throats, should be grappled with in every possible way, first by gargling with the remedy pure, second by filling each car with the remedy pure, one after the other, and letting it remain in each ear ten minutes. I have found great relief from this method, and the. best time is upon retiring to rest. Then a little linen, saturated with the remedy, should be wrapped round the neck, and kept moist; these methods are generally successful; but if not the danger from the sore throat becoming something worse is greatly reduced.

This is one of those complaints which re?uire great perseverance, and even the use of leeches may be necessary after all; but such eases will be very rare.

INFLAMMATION in the Bowels is cured by taking two table-spoonsful of the remedy, diluted with hot water, repeatedly, and at short intervals, until the. pain is removed. It is. also well to rub the exterior, and apply warm flannel to the part, which may be kept warm, or even hot, by applying a warming pan to the flannel.

Pains in the Side, which are often the forerunners of Pleurisies and other Fevers. After the crown of the head has been rubbed, the side should be well rubbed with the remedy until the pain is re- moved. If this does not succeed, it will be necessary to take a piece, of linen, about half a yard square, and double it several times, until it becomes six inches square; saturate it well with the remedy, and apply it to the part ; it should be kept moist. It has been of great use in numberless instances, and generally removes the pain in less than an hour, and very often prevents fever. It will also be well for the patient to take two table-spoonsful of the remedy, diluted with hot water.

Rheumatism is always relieved, and often cured, by rubbing with this remedy upon the part afflicted. But it ought to be continued for several days, or even weeks, once or twice each day, and there are cases in which it is necessary the patient should take two table-spoonsful, mixed with hot water, once a day, for twelve or four- teen days. This is one of the most stubborn complaints in existence, and requires great patience and perseverance; but even this has been obliged to yield to tbc remedy, though the use of a brush is sometimes necessary.

A great many instances might be adduced of persons afflicted with this complaint who have been obliged to pass their winters, in great pain, within doors, but by its application have been able to enjoy themselves during the whole of the year.

Gout and Rheumatic Gout. — These painful disorders being in the blood, it will be necessary that the person afflicted should have his or her crown of the head well rubbed with the remedy, once, on retiring to rest; the morning after take two table-spoonsful mixed with hot water, an hour before breakfast, which should be repeated for twelve or fourteen days, and the part inflamed, or where the pain is, touched with something soft, perhaps a feather, until the patient can bear to rub it with the finger.

These are complaints which re?uire great perseverance.

Gravel. — Take a table-spoonful (diluted) three or four times a day.

Burns and Scalds are very soon cured by tins remedy. The part afTected should be rubbed with the pure liquid. The first application is painful, but not of long continuance, and each application is less painful. The sore is soon cured, but sometimes it is necessary to apply something to soften the sore; tallow or hog's lard is good, or anything else of a softening nature.

Chilblains are cured by the application of this remedy; but care should be taken that the part affected should be rubbed until perfectly dry. There is also another cure, which is simply washing the hands or feet in a strong ley of salt and water, and let it dry upon them.

Insanity, or what is called Affection of the Nerves, which produces lowness of spirits, may be almost always prevented by rubbing the crown of the head twice or thrice with this remedy. But it ought to be well rubbed each time for ten minutes, or a quarter of an hour; and I think, in order to confirm the cure, two table-spoonsful should be taken for twelve mornings, tasting, diluted with hot water.

Children of the age of four years, and under, are cured by rubbing the crown of the head only once. I have had so many proofs of it that I can speak with great confidence. There is only one case in which it was not successful, and that was an eruption on the skin; in all other complaints, whether illness or weakness, it has been successful.

CANCERS. — I have had such great success in the cure of them that I thought, it never failed, and that merely by rubbing or washing the sore. There are at present some doubts whether it cures those of a very long standing or not, but there is not the least doubt that it will cure those which have been in existence for a year, and it may be easily known whether the sore is of a cancerous nature or not by the application of the remedy. If it is so, the application gives no pain, and the cure is rapid ; to all other sores it gives pain.

For cancers of long standing, I recommend that the crown of the head should be well rubbed with the remedy, and that the. patient should take two table-spoonsful, diluted with hot water every morning. The sore ought to be washed with the remedy, and soft linen saturated with the remedy applied, and kept, if possible, constantly it. In all cases, if this method is followed, it will be a great relief, and generally a cure; ami, for the future, there will be very few bad cancers, if the remedy is applied in their early stage.

"Worms. — Take two table-spoonsful of the remedy pure, an hour before breakfast; for a child, from five to seven years of age, half the quantity is sufficient.

Fevers. — In all cases of fexcr, and there are several kinds, rubbing the crown of the head with the remedy should he the very first operation, and immediately after the patient should take two table- spoonsful, diluted with hot water; this should be repeated at intervals of from an hour to three hours, according to the nature acid violence of the attack. No amendment can be hoped for until the inflammation is reduced, and nothing will reduce it so soon as this remedy, and that without bleeding and blistering; but all complaints are the most easily cured at their commencement.

Inflammation on the Lungs will generally be relieved by washing the crown of the head, and taking two table-spoonsful, diluted with hot water. But it should be taken'several times each day, and a piece of linen, several thicknesses, saturated with the remedy, put upon the part where the pain is.

Consumptions. — I have not the least doubt but the majority might be cured by an application of this remedy, in its earlier stages, and that without confinement, by first rubbing the crown of the head once, and taking one or two table-spoonsful of the remedy, diluted with hot water, every morning, an hour before breakfast; it will be well to rub the chest once each morning. There are two cases of its almost wonderful effects, one at La Ferte Imbault, and the other in the* Isle of Man. *

As the remedy is a new discovery, the cases of its cure of this complaint are not many; but only let it be properly and generally used, and I have no doubt but millions will derive benefit from it each year.

Asthmas are greatly relieved by rubbing the crown of the head once, before retiring to rest, and taking one or two table-spoonsful diluted with hot water, for several mornings.

Colds and Coughs are greatly relieved by the application of this remedy to the parts affected. If in the head, the head should be rubbed; if in the throat, the ears should be filled, one after the other, and let remain for ten minutes, the throat gargled, and the neck and breast rubbed with the remedy. They are oft very tedious, and re?uire great perseverance, and even with all this it is ne-

Brandy and Salt. — (a mixture of brandy and salt) strongly recom-mended by its discoverer, as a powerful remedy in several dangerous mala- dies which afflict the human race.

Dysentery, if violent, should be (rented by rubbing the crown of the bead with the remedy once, and immediately taking one or two table-spoonsful diluted with hot water; this should be repeated three or four times each day. The disorder must be very bad if it is not subdued in two or three days; but perseverance is necessary.

Sprains are easily cured with this remedy; sometimes by merely rubbing ; but if that does not succeed, by taking a long piece of linen, about two inches' broad, and wrapping it several times round the part, after it has been saturated with the remedy, they are generally cured in a day or two ; but the linen should be kept moist with the remedy the whole of the time, until a cure is effected.

Bruisks sometimes require to be several times nibbed with the remedy. At other times once or twice suffices: but it is always well to persevere until the cure is effected. The application "fives no pain; but sometimes bruises are rather tedious in being cured.

Scurvy only re?uires to be rubbed with the remedy several times until the complaint is subdued. But if the person afflicted considers his blood to be any way bad, he will do well to have the crown of the head rubbed with the remedy, and take one or two table-spoonsful, diluted with hot water, each morning before breakfast, for twelve mornings. It will generally purify the blood in that time.

Itch, I believe, may be cured by this remedy, by washing or rub- bing with it till the complaint is subdued. But this is often tedious, and re?uires perseverance and great cleanliness.

Ring-Worms, upon children's heads, are easily cured by rubbing the bead with the remedy. It very seldom takes a week to cure the complaint, and nothing can be done which conduces more to the general health of children than rubbing the head. Many schools are broken up by this teasing complaint, which might be avoided by the master or mistress using it for the children. 1 believe its infecting ?ualities are removed by the first application.

Paralytic Attacks should be attended to the same moment as the attack commences; and this will show the necessity of all families being provided with a bottle ready prepared. The crown of the head should be well rubbed with the remedy, and at the same time the patient should have two table-spoonsful for a woman, and three table-spoonsful for a man given, diluted with hot water. Another person ought to be employed in rubbing the part affected with the remedy. Perhaps it may be necessary to give the patient more than one dose; but this must be left to the discretion of his friends. It is sure to do good in repeating it.

Pregnancy. — Pregnant women ought to take one table-spoonful diluted with hot water, once a week or fortnight, but not oftener, during their pregnancy. It renders the child more healthy, and the delivery is effected with greater ease.

Bites of Poisonous Reptiles are easily cured by rubbing the parts bitten with the remedy. It neutralises the poison, and heals the sore in a very short time; but it is well to do it immediately after the bite has been given.

Bites of Mad Dogs, or any other dogs, are easily cured by rubbing well the part bitten with this remedy. I believe no uneasiness may be felt by the person bitten, if it is rubbed the same day; but it is always best to do it immediately after, and it ought to be rubbed several times, and a piece of soft linen, saturated with the remedy, applied to the part.

Stings of Wasps, Bees, &c., are cured by rubbing the part immediately after being stung"; the relief, as well as the attack, is instantaneous; but I do not think it does much good if the part is suffered to swell ; therefore the application should be prompt.

Erisipelas is cured by rubbing the part with the remedy.

Tic Doloreux. — This painfnl complaint may be. greatly relieved by the use of this remedy; perhaps cured if it is in the face. The crown of the head should be well rubbed with the remedy; after which the ear on the side of the head next it should be filled with the remedy, which should remain in for ten minutes. After, the part affected should be rubbed with the remedy. If these fail of effecting a cure, I should recommend that the patient should take two table-spoonsful of the remedy, diluted with hot water, each morning before breakfast, about an hour, for fourteen days.

Scrofula must be very difficult to cure; but as it is in the blood, that ought to be purified, which is easily effected, by first rubbing the crown of the head once with the remedy, after which the patient should take one or two table-spoonsful of the remedy, diluted with hot water, an hour before breakfast, every morning for at least a month; and the sores should be covered with soft linen, saturated with the remedy. It will also be well to apply something softening to the sore.

Bilious Complaints are cured by rubbing first the crown of the head once before retiring to rest, and next morning taking two table-spoonsful of the remedy diluted with hot water, an hour before breakfast, for twenty mornings. Before half of that time is passed the good effects of the application will be seen in the face of the patient, which, from sickly yellow or white, will become fair and ruddy. But this is a small part of the benefit, as the afflicted will acknowledge.

Bites of Mus?uitoes, Gnats, and other Noxious Insects, may be cured by only rubbing the part bitten with the remedy.

Plague, being an inflammatory complaint, I hope may be cured, by the same method as others of the same description; that is, by first rubbing the crown of the head, and immediately after giving the patient three table-spoonsful, diluted with hot water, which ought to be lepeated every ten minutes, if the patient can take it, until the complaint is subdued.

Mortification is almost as easily stopped, and the cure effected, It was applied as to any common sore, by wrapping a piece of soft linen, saturated with the remedy, upon the sore and kept humid, by wetting it several times a day.

Boils and Abscesses should be covered with a piece of soft linen, saturated with the remedy, and kept wet. By this means though it does not prevent or retard the bursting of the boil or abscess, it very much relieves the pain by removing the inflammation.

Cuts. — As a tincture, I do not think that this remedy has its e?ual, giving very little pain when first applied, and curing in a short time. Any person will know that the application should be made by saturating a piece of linen in the remdey, and wrapping it round the part cut, which must be very severe if there is occasion to remove, the linen till the cure is effected. But it should be kept always moist by adding a little of the remedy several times each day.

Whitlow may be cured by either holding the finger in the remedy, or saturating a piece of soft linen with it, and wrapping it round the sore. But it should be kept wet until the cure is effected.

Lumbago, though comprised under the head of Rheumatism, it is well to observe, is generally removed by rubbing the part. But if it cannot be removed by that means, or it returns again, 1 should recommend the patient to have the crown of the head well rubbed once, on retiring to rest, with the remedy, and then taking, for several mornings, an hour before breakfast, two table-spoonsful of the remedy, diluted with hot water.

Jaundice, I believe, may be cured by rubbing the crown of the head once, on retiring to rest, and taking two table-spoonsful, diluted with hot water, for several mornings, an hour before breakfast, until the complaint disappears, which I expect it will do in eight or ten days.

Liver Complaints and Affections of the Heart can only be removed by putting the intestines in a healthful state, which may be effected by rubbing the crown of the head once, on retiring to rest, and each morning taking two table-spoonsful of the remedy, diluted with hot water, an hour before breakfast; perhaps it re?uires to be taken for months before the complaints are cured. But prevention is always better than cure, therefore the intestines should be kept healthy, and the blood pure.

Sores of long standing are relieved, and very often cured, by this remedy, by saturating soft linen with it, and applying it to the sore. After three or four applications it always relieves the pain; and the most obstinate setfasts are removed, and that without pain, in a few days, and the sore becomes clean, not only from that, but all other impurities. How many poor creatures pass lives of misery from incurable sores, who will be relieved by the use of this remedy!

There are many instances of persons who have not been able to sleep for weeks, who have slept the very first night after its application; and all, let their case be ever so bad, may have the same consolation if they apply this simple remedy.

Yellow Fever, which often terminates in the Black Fever, called the Black Vomit, is, I suppose, much of the same nature as the Plague; therefore it must be treated in the same manner. 1 have no doubt but a great many lives may be preserved by that method.

Gall Stones are no doubt produced by the intestines being in an unhealthy state: therefore it is well to keep them always healthy, which may be generally effected by rubbing the crown of the head once, and taking the remedy, each morning for a week or ten days, an hour before breakfast, diluted with hot water. A beloved sister suffered, and was confined to bed, for several months, by refusing to use it as above. After the Gall Stones are formed, I do not think they can be removed by any other than the ordinary method, but the pain may be greatly alleviated by the application of this remedy; the pain ought to be attacked in every possible way, by rubbing the exterior, and applying fomentations to the part nearest the pain.

Indigestion may be easily corrected by rubbing the crown of the head once, and taking one or two table-spoonsful of the remedy, diluted with hot water, every morning, until the complaint is removed; as a corrective, this remedy is very efficacious.

Spinal Complaints, I believe, have their source in the head ; therefore it will be well first to rub the crown of the head with the remedy, on retiring to rest, after which, next morning, the patient should take one or two table-spoonsful of the remedy, diluted with hot water, an hour before breakfast, each morning, for twelve mornings, or till the complaint is removed. Soft linen, of several thicknesses, saturated with the remedy, should be applied to the part where the pain is, if rubbing does not remove it, and it should be renewed several times a day if the spine is very painful, and always kept moist. Application, in this manner, for two or three days, is sure to reduce the pain, though it may not cure the complaint so soon.

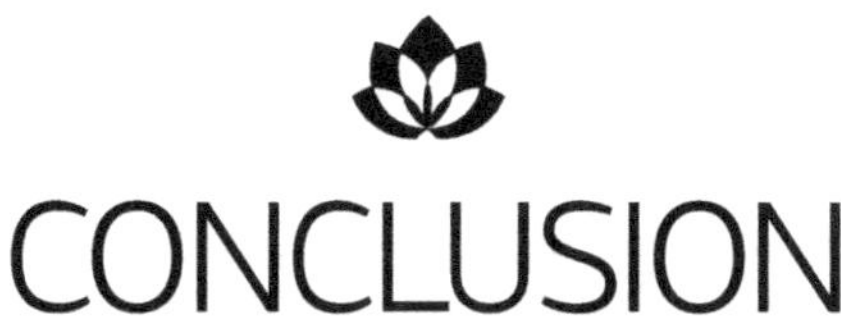

CHAPTER EIGHT

CONCLUSION

In conclusion, I beg leave to say, that as a remedy it is unrivalled; whether it is used internally or externally, it is equally efficacious, and for both, or either, there cannot be found its e?ual; therefore, as a remedy, it is almost perfect. As a discovery I cannot but think it stands unrivalled also, at least in medicine, as there is nothing made public which is equal to it as an universal specific. It cures complaints which have hitherto been deemed incurable.

This has been thought to be an objection to it; but let these objectors apply it according to the rules laid down in this treatise, and I think they will blush at their want of caution. As a remedy, which is easily made, I do think it cannot be exceeded; all that is wanted is to apply a sufficient ?uantity of salt to the brandy, shake it together, and it is ready for use as soon as it is clear.

This is no alternative for serious medical treatment and should be taken only under medical control...